# ATKINS DIET FOR BEGINNERS

By

**DR. JULIE OWENS**

Contents

# Chapter 1

## INTRODUCTION TO THE ATKINS DIET

## 1. What is the Atkins diet?

The Atkins diet is a low-carbohydrate diet that emphasizes protein and fats while limiting the intake of carbohydrates. It was created by Dr. Robert Atkins in the 1970s and gained popularity for its potential to aid in weight loss and improve overall health. The diet typically consists of four phases:

**Induction phase:** This phase is the most restrictive, limiting carbohydrate intake to around 20 grams per day, primarily from vegetables. Protein, fats, and non-starchy vegetables are encouraged.

**Balancing phase:** During this phase, carbohydrate intake is gradually increased in 5-gram increments each week, focusing on finding the individual's "critical carbohydrate level for losing weight" (CCLL) where weight loss occurs without hunger.

**Fine-tuning phase:** Once near the weight goal, the dieter enters this phase to fine-tune carbohydrate intake to maintain weight loss.

**Maintenance phase:** In this phase, the dieter can consume more carbohydrates as long as weight maintenance is achieved.

The Atkins diet aims to shift the body's metabolism from burning carbohydrates for energy to burning stored fat, known as ketosis. This process is similar to the ketogenic diet, but the Atkins diet allows for more flexibility in carbohydrate intake as the dieter progresses through the phases. It is important to note that while the Atkins diet can be effective for some individuals in weight loss and managing blood sugar levels, it may not be suitable for everyone, and consulting with a healthcare provider is recommended before starting any new diet plan.

## 2. History and evolution of the Atkins diet

The Atkins diet, also known as the Atkins Nutritional Approach, is a low-carbohydrate diet created by Dr. Robert Atkins in the 1970s. The diet gained popularity for its focus on limiting carbohydrates and promoting high-protein and high-fat foods. Here's a brief history and evolution of the Atkins diet:

**1972:** Dr. Robert Atkins publishes his book "Dr. Atkins' Diet Revolution," which introduces his low-carbohydrate approach to weight loss. The diet emphasizes reducing carbohydrates while allowing unlimited protein and fat intake.

**1992:** Dr. Atkins releases an updated version of his book titled "Dr. Atkins' New Diet Revolution," which further popularizes the Atkins diet. This edition includes more detailed guidelines and meal plans.

**2002:** The Atkins Nutritional Approach undergoes a significant update with the release of "Dr. Atkins' New Diet Revolution," which introduces the concept of "Net Carbs." Net Carbs are calculated by subtracting fiber and sugar alcohols from the total carbohydrate content of foods, with the belief that these types of carbohydrates have a minimal impact on blood sugar levels.

**2003:** The popularity of the Atkins diet peaks, with many people adopting it for weight loss and improved health.

However, critics raise concerns about its high saturated fat intake and potential long-term health risks.

**2007:** Dr. Atkins Nutritionals, Inc. files for bankruptcy due to declining sales and legal issues. The company is later acquired by North Castle Partners, a private equity firm.

**2010s:** The Atkins diet evolves to address some of the criticisms by promoting a more balanced approach to nutrition. The emphasis shifts towards whole foods, healthy fats, and lean proteins, with less focus on processed foods and saturated fats.

**Present:** The Atkins diet continues to be a popular choice for individuals looking to lose weight or manage their carbohydrate intake. It has inspired variations and spin-offs, such as the "Modified Atkins Diet" for epilepsy treatment and the "Eco-Atkins Diet," which is a plant-based version focusing on vegetable proteins.

Throughout its history, the Atkins diet has sparked debates among health professionals and researchers regarding its effectiveness, safety, and long-term sustainability. While some studies suggest that it can lead to significant weight loss and improvements in certain health markers, others raise concerns about potential risks associated with high-fat and high-protein diets. As with any diet, individual results and experiences can vary, and it's important to consult with a healthcare provider before making significant dietary changes.

# 3. Basic principles and philosophy behind the Atkins diet

**Carbohydrate restriction:** The Atkins diet focuses on limiting carbohydrate intake to shift the body's metabolism from using glucose (from carbohydrates) as its primary fuel source to using stored fat for energy. This is known as a state of ketosis.

**Phases: The diet is divided into four phases:**

**Induction phase:** This initial phase restricts carbohydrate intake to 20-25 grams per day for two weeks to jumpstart weight loss and transition the body into ketosis.

**Balancing phase:** This phase gradually adds more carbohydrates back into the diet, focusing on nutrient-dense, low-glycemic index foods to find the individual's carbohydrate tolerance level for weight maintenance or continued weight loss.

**Fine-tuning phase:** Once close to the goal weight, carbohydrates are further increased to find the ideal long-term carbohydrate intake for weight maintenance.

**Maintenance phase:** In this final phase, individuals can consume a higher level of carbohydrates while still maintaining their weight loss or weight maintenance goals.

**Protein and fat:** The Atkins diet encourages the consumption of protein and healthy fats, such as avocados, nuts, seeds, and olive oil, to provide satiety and essential nutrients.

**Vegetable and fiber intake:** Non-starchy vegetables are encouraged in all phases of the diet, providing fiber and essential nutrients while contributing fewer carbohydrates.

**Emphasis on whole foods:** The Atkins diet promotes whole, unprocessed foods and discourages processed and refined carbohydrates and sugars.

**Individualized approach:** The diet allows for customization based on individual needs and goals, with the ability to adjust carbohydrate intake to suit lifestyle and health goals.

## 4. Different phases of the Atkins diet (Induction, Ongoing Weight Loss, Pre-Maintenance, Maintenance)

**Induction Phase:** This phase is the most restrictive and is designed to kickstart weight loss by transitioning the body into a state of ketosis, where it burns fat for fuel instead of carbohydrates. During this phase, which typically lasts for about two weeks, carbohydrate intake is limited to 20-25 grams per day, mostly coming from non-starchy vegetables. Foods like meat, fish, eggs, cheese, and fats are encouraged. This phase is meant to jumpstart weight loss and reduce cravings for sugary and starchy foods.

**Ongoing Weight Loss (OWL) Phase:** In this phase, you gradually increase your carbohydrate intake by 5 grams per week, aiming to find your personal carbohydrate tolerance level where you continue to lose weight steadily. This phase allows for a wider variety of foods, including more vegetables, nuts, and low-carb fruits. You continue this phase until you are 10 pounds from your goal weight.

**Pre-Maintenance Phase:** This phase helps you prepare for maintenance by gradually increasing your carbohydrate intake by 10 grams per week. You continue to monitor your weight and adjust your carb intake until you reach your goal weight. This phase helps prevent weight regain by slowly reintroducing carbs and finding the right balance for weight maintenance.

**Maintenance Phase:** Once you've reached your goal weight, you enter the maintenance phase, where you can increase your carb intake further if your weight remains stable. The goal is to find the maximum amount of carbs you can eat without gaining weight. This phase emphasizes a balanced diet with a focus on whole foods, healthy fats, and adequate protein.

## 5. Benefits and potential drawbacks of the Atkins diet

> **Benefits:**

**Weight loss:** The Atkins diet restricts carbohydrates, which can lead to rapid weight loss, especially in the initial phase.

**Appetite control:** High-protein and high-fat foods can help you feel full and satisfied, reducing overall calorie intake.

**Improved blood sugar control:** By limiting carbohydrates, the Atkins diet can help stabilize blood sugar levels, which is beneficial for people with diabetes or insulin resistance.

**Triglyceride levels:** Some studies suggest that the Atkins diet may lower triglyceride levels, which is beneficial for heart health.

**HDL cholesterol:** The diet may also increase levels of high-density lipoprotein (HDL) cholesterol, which is known as the "good" cholesterol.

➢ **Drawbacks:**

**Nutrient deficiencies:** The Atkins diet restricts many foods that are rich in essential nutrients, such as fruits, whole grains, and certain vegetables, which can lead to deficiencies if not carefully planned.

**Constipation:** The low-fiber nature of the diet can lead to constipation for some people, especially if they don't consume enough vegetables or fiber supplements.

**Ketosis:** The Atkins diet can induce a state of ketosis, where the body burns fat for fuel instead of carbohydrates. While this can lead to rapid weight loss, it can also cause side effects such as bad breath, fatigue, and nausea.

**Long-term sustainability:** Some people find the strict carbohydrate restrictions of the Atkins diet difficult to maintain over the long term, leading to weight regain once they resume a more typical diet.

# Chapter 2

## GETTING STARTED WITH THE ATKINS DIET

## 1. Preparing for the Atkins diet (consulting with healthcare professionals, setting realistic goals)

**Consult with Healthcare Professionals:** Before starting any new diet, including the Atkins diet, it's essential to consult with a healthcare professional, such as a doctor or a registered dietitian. They can provide personalized guidance based on your health status, dietary needs, and any underlying medical conditions.

**Set Realistic Goals:** Set clear, achievable goals for your Atkins diet journey. These goals should be specific, measurable, attainable, relevant, and time-bound (SMART). Examples of goals might include losing a certain amount of weight, improving blood sugar levels, or increasing energy levels.

**Educate Yourself:** Take the time to understand the basic principles and philosophy behind the Atkins diet. This includes learning about the different phases of the diet, the role of carbohydrates, protein, and fats, and how the diet may impact your body.

**Plan Your Meals:** Create a meal plan that aligns with the Atkins diet principles. This involves understanding which foods are allowed in each phase of the diet, how to balance your macronutrients (carbohydrates, protein, and fat), and incorporating a variety of foods to ensure you're getting essential nutrients.

**Monitor Your Progress:** Keep track of your progress on the Atkins diet. This can include tracking your weight, body measurements, energy levels, and any changes in health markers (like blood sugar levels, if applicable). This information can help you adjust your diet and goals as needed.

**Stay Flexible and Adapt:** While it's important to have a plan, be prepared to adapt it based on your body's response and your personal preferences. The Atkins diet offers different phases, so you can adjust your carbohydrate intake based on how your body reacts and your specific goals.

## 2. Understanding macronutrients (carbohydrates, proteins, fats) and their role in the Atkins diet

**Carbohydrates:** In the Atkins diet, carbohydrates are limited, especially in the initial phase called the "Induction Phase." This phase typically restricts carbohydrate intake to 20-25 grams per day to induce a state of ketosis, where the body switches from using carbohydrates as its primary source of fuel to burning stored fat for energy. As you progress through the diet, you gradually increase your carbohydrate intake in later phases while still maintaining a level that allows you to continue losing or maintaining weight.

**Proteins:** Protein is an important component of the Atkins diet, as it helps maintain muscle mass and supports satiety. During the Induction Phase and subsequent phases, you're encouraged to consume moderate amounts of protein from sources like meat, poultry, fish, eggs, and tofu. The diet emphasizes lean protein choices to minimize saturated fat intake.

**Fats:** The Atkins diet promotes the consumption of healthy fats, including monounsaturated and polyunsaturated fats, while limiting trans fats and saturated fats. Healthy fat sources include avocados, nuts, seeds, olive oil, and fatty fish. Fats are an essential part of the diet because they provide energy and help you feel full, which can aid in weight loss by reducing overall calorie intake.

## 3. Grocery shopping and meal planning tips for the Atkins diet

**Protein:** Include plenty of protein-rich foods like chicken, turkey, beef, pork, fish, seafood, eggs, and tofu.

**Low-carb vegetables:** Choose non-starchy vegetables like spinach, kale, broccoli, cauliflower, bell peppers, zucchini, asparagus, and mushrooms.

**Healthy fats:** Opt for sources of healthy fats such as avocado, olive oil, coconut oil, nuts (almonds, walnuts, pecans), and seeds (flaxseeds, chia seeds).

**Dairy:** Select full-fat dairy products like cheese, yogurt, and cream.

**Low-carb snacks:** Look for snacks that are low in carbs and high in protein, such as beef jerky, pork rinds, cheese sticks, and nuts.

> ➢ **For meal planning:**

**Balanced meals:** Aim for meals that include a protein source, healthy fats, and non-starchy vegetables. For example, grilled chicken with a side of sautéed spinach and avocado.

**Snacks:** Plan for snacks that are low in carbs but satisfying, like cheese and nuts or veggies with dip.

**Variety:** Keep your meals interesting by trying different protein sources and vegetables. Experiment with different spices and herbs for flavor.

**Preparation:** Consider preparing meals in advance to have healthy options readily available. This can help you stick to your diet plan even on busy days.

**Hydration:** Stay hydrated by drinking plenty of water throughout the day. Sometimes thirst can be mistaken for hunger.

## 4.Sample meal plans for each phase of the Atkins diet

> **Phase 1: Induction**

**Breakfast:** Scrambled eggs with spinach and cheese cooked in butter

**Snack:** Celery sticks with cream cheese

**Lunch:** Grilled chicken breast with mixed greens and olive oil dressing

**Snack:** Turkey slices rolled with cheese

**Dinner:** Baked salmon with steamed broccoli and butter

> **Phase 2: Balancing**

**Breakfast:** Greek yogurt with berries and nuts

**Snack:** Cottage cheese with cucumber slices

**Lunch:** Turkey and avocado lettuce wraps

**Snack:** Almonds

**Dinner:** Grilled steak with asparagus and a side salad

> **Phase 3: Fine-Tuning**

**Breakfast:** Omelette with mushrooms, peppers, and cheese

**Snack:** Apple slices with almond butter

**Lunch:** Tuna salad with mixed greens

**Snack:** Cheese and pepperoni slices

**Dinner:** Stir-fried shrimp with vegetables in coconut oil

> **Phase 4: Maintenance**

**Breakfast:** Smoothie with spinach, berries, protein powder, and almond milk

**Snack:** Carrot sticks with hummus

**Lunch:** Grilled chicken Caesar salad

**Snack:** Hard-boiled eggs

**Dinner:** Baked cod with roasted Brussels sprouts and a side of quinoa

# Chapter 3

## THE INDUCTION PHASE

## 1. Overview of the Induction phase (duration, carbohydrate restriction)

**Duration:** The Induction phase typically lasts for two weeks, but it can vary based on individual goals and needs. Some people may choose to stay in this phase longer if they have more weight to lose or if they find it effective for managing their carbohydrate cravings.

**Carbohydrate Restriction:** During the Induction phase, carbohydrate intake is limited to 20-25 grams of net carbs per day. Net carbs are calculated by subtracting fiber and sugar alcohols (if applicable) from the total carbohydrate content of a food.

**Focus on Protein and Fat:** To compensate for the reduction in carbs, the diet emphasizes protein-rich foods such as meat, poultry, fish, and eggs, as well as healthy fats like olive oil, avocado, and nuts.

**Transitioning into Ketosis:** By restricting carbohydrates, the body is forced to use its stored fat for energy, a state known as ketosis. This can lead to rapid weight loss, especially in the form of water weight in the initial stages.

**Possible Side Effects:** Some people may experience side effects during the Induction phase, such as fatigue, dizziness, headaches, or irritability. These symptoms are often temporary and can be managed by staying hydrated, getting enough electrolytes, and ensuring an adequate intake of vitamins and minerals.

**Monitoring Progress:** It's important to track your progress during the Induction phase by monitoring your weight, energy levels, and how you feel overall. This can help you determine if the diet is working for you and if any adjustments need to be made.

**Consultation with Healthcare Professionals:** Before starting the Atkins diet or any other low-carb diet, it's advisable to consult with a healthcare professional, especially if you have any underlying health conditions or are taking medication.

# 2. Allowed foods during the Induction phase (low-carb vegetables, protein sources, fats)

➢ **Low-carb vegetables:**

Leafy greens (e.g., spinach, kale, lettuce)

Cruciferous vegetables (e.g., broccoli, cauliflower, Brussels sprouts)

Zucchini

Bell peppers

Cucumber

Celery

Asparagus

Eggplant

Tomatoes (in moderation)

➢ **Protein sources:**

Meat (beef, pork, lamb, chicken, turkey)

Fish (salmon, trout, sardines, mackerel)

Shellfish (shrimp, crab, lobster)

Eggs

Tofu and other soy products (in moderation)

> **Fats:**

Butter

Olive oil

Coconut oil

Avocado oil

Lard

Ghee

## 3. Tips for managing potential side effects (carb withdrawal, keto flu)

**Stay Hydrated:** Drink plenty of water to help flush out toxins and reduce the risk of dehydration, which can worsen symptoms.

**Electrolytes:** Replace electrolytes lost through increased urination by consuming foods rich in potassium, magnesium, and sodium or using supplements.

**Gradual Reduction:** If possible, gradually reduce your carbohydrate intake over a few weeks before starting the diet to help minimize withdrawal symptoms.

**Eat Enough Fat and Protein:** Ensure you're getting enough healthy fats and protein to help keep you satiated and maintain energy levels.

**Include Fiber:** Consume fiber-rich foods like vegetables, nuts, and seeds to aid digestion and promote a feeling of fullness.

**Rest and Sleep:** Get plenty of rest to help your body adjust to the diet and reduce fatigue.

**Manage Stress:** Stress can exacerbate symptoms, so practice stress-reducing activities like meditation, yoga, or deep breathing exercises.

**Exercise:** Light exercise can help boost your mood and energy levels, but avoid intense workouts during the initial phase of the diet.

**Consider Supplements:** Talk to your healthcare provider about supplements like B vitamins, vitamin D, and omega-3 fatty acids to support overall health during the diet.

**Be Patient:** Remember that these side effects are temporary and usually subside within a few days to a week as your body adjusts to the diet.

## 4. Tracking progress and adjusting the diet during the Induction phase

**Track Your Carbohydrate Intake:** Keep a daily record of the number of grams of carbohydrates you consume. The

Induction phase limits your carbohydrate intake to about 20 grams per day, mostly from vegetables.

**Monitor Your Weight:** Weigh yourself regularly (e.g., once a week) to track your weight loss progress. Remember that weight loss can vary from person to person.

**Check Your Ketone Levels:** The Induction phase aims to induce a state of ketosis, where your body burns fat for fuel. You can use ketone test strips to monitor your ketone levels. The presence of ketones indicates that you are in ketosis.

**Assess Your Energy Levels and Hunger:** Pay attention to how you feel throughout the day. If you feel excessively tired or hungry, you may need to adjust your food intake or meal timing.

**Adjust Your Macronutrient Ratios:** If you're not seeing the desired results, you may need to adjust your macronutrient ratios. For example, you may need to increase your fat intake and decrease your protein intake.

**Stay Hydrated:** Drink plenty of water to stay hydrated, especially since the Induction phase can cause water loss due to lower carbohydrate intake.

**Consult with a Healthcare Professional:** If you have any concerns or are unsure about how to adjust your diet, it's best to consult with a healthcare professional or a registered dietitian who can provide personalized advice based on your individual needs and goals.

# Chapter 4

## THE ONGOING WEIGHT LOSS PHASE

## 1.Transitioning from the Induction phase to the Ongoing Weight Loss phase

**Gradual Carb Increase:** In the OWL phase, you gradually increase your carb intake in 5-gram increments each week. This helps you find your personal carb tolerance level, where you continue to lose weight but maintain good energy levels.

**Choose the Right Carbs:** Focus on nutrient-dense, high-fiber carbs like vegetables, nuts, seeds, and berries. Avoid refined carbs and sugars, as they can cause blood sugar spikes and cravings.

**Monitor Your Progress:** Keep track of your weight, energy levels, and how you feel after eating different amounts of carbs. This will help you determine the right carb level for you.

**Stay Hydrated:** Drink plenty of water, as it helps with digestion and can prevent constipation, which can sometimes occur when increasing carbs.

**Continue with Protein:** Protein should still be a cornerstone of your meals, as it helps you feel full and supports muscle maintenance.

**Healthy Fats:** Include healthy fats like olive oil, avocados, and nuts in your diet. They provide energy and help you feel satisfied.

**Regular Exercise:** Physical activity is important for overall health and can enhance weight loss. Aim for a combination of cardio and strength training.

**Mindful Eating:** Pay attention to your hunger and fullness cues. Stop eating when you're satisfied, not stuffed.

**Plan Your Meals:** Meal planning can help you stay on track and make healthy choices.

**Seek Support:** Joining a community or finding a buddy who is also following the Atkins diet can provide motivation and accountability.

## 2. Balancing carbohydrate intake with ongoing weight loss goals

**Monitor Your Carb Intake:** Continue tracking your daily carbohydrate intake to ensure you're within your carb limit for ongoing weight loss. Gradually increase your carb intake in 5-gram increments each week until you find your personal carb balance, where you continue to lose weight.

**Choose Low-Carb Foods:** Focus on low-carb, high-fiber vegetables, and nutrient-dense foods. Avoid refined carbs and sugars as much as possible.

**Include Healthy Fats and Proteins:** Healthy fats and proteins should still make up a significant portion of your diet. They help keep you satisfied and provide essential nutrients.

**Meal Planning:** Plan your meals ahead of time to ensure they are balanced and within your carb limit. This can help prevent impulsive food choices.

**Stay Active:** Regular physical activity can help support your weight loss goals and overall health.

**Stay Hydrated:** Drink plenty of water throughout the day, as dehydration can sometimes be mistaken for hunger.

**Listen to Your Body:** Pay attention to how different foods affect your body and adjust your diet accordingly.

# 3. Incorporating more variety into the diet while maintaining low-carb principles

**Explore Different Vegetables:** Try new low-carb vegetables like kale, spinach, broccoli, cauliflower, zucchini, bell peppers, and asparagus. These can be roasted, grilled, sautéed, or enjoyed raw in salads.

**Experiment with Proteins:** Include a variety of proteins such as poultry, fish, seafood, eggs, and tofu. Try different cooking methods like baking, grilling, or stir-frying for variety.

**Incorporate Healthy Fats:** Include sources of healthy fats like avocados, nuts, seeds, and olive oil. These can add flavor and richness to your meals.

**Use Herbs and Spices:** Experiment with different herbs and spices to enhance the flavor of your dishes without adding carbs. Cumin, paprika, turmeric, and garlic can add depth to your meals.

**Try Low-Carb Substitutes:** Explore low-carb alternatives to your favorite high-carb foods, such as cauliflower rice or zucchini noodles in place of rice or pasta.

**Include Dairy in Moderation:** Dairy products like cheese, yogurt, and cream can add variety to your meals, but be mindful of their carb content and choose full-fat options.

**Plan Balanced Meals:** Aim for a balance of protein, healthy fats, and vegetables in each meal to ensure you're getting a variety of nutrients.

**Explore Ethnic Cuisines:** Many ethnic cuisines offer low-carb options, such as Mexican fajitas without the tortillas, or Japanese sashimi and cucumber rolls.

**Get Creative with Recipes:** Look for low-carb recipes online or in cookbooks for inspiration. There are many creative ways to enjoy a variety of flavors while keeping carbs in check.

**Listen to Your Body:** Pay attention to how different foods make you feel. Everyone's tolerance for carbs can vary, so adjust your diet based on how your body responds.

## 4. Tips for staying motivated and overcoming plateaus during this phase

**Set Realistic Goals:** Review your weight loss goals and make sure they are realistic and achievable. Break them down into smaller, manageable targets.

**Track Your Progress:** Keep track of your weight loss, measurements, and how you feel. This can help you stay motivated and see how far you've come.

**Mix Up Your Meals:** Try new recipes and foods to keep your meals exciting and prevent boredom. This can help you stick to your low-carb diet plan.

**Stay Active:** Regular physical activity can help boost your metabolism and break through plateaus. Incorporate a mix of cardio and strength training exercises into your routine.

**Stay Hydrated:** Drinking plenty of water can help you feel full and prevent overeating. It can also help with digestion and overall health.

**Get Enough Sleep:** Lack of sleep can affect your weight loss efforts. Aim for 7-9 hours of quality sleep per night to support your overall health and well-being.

**Manage Stress:** Stress can impact your weight loss journey. Find healthy ways to manage stress, such as meditation, yoga, or deep breathing exercises.

**Consult with a Healthcare Professional:** If you're struggling to overcome a plateau, consider consulting with a healthcare professional or a registered dietitian. They can provide personalized advice and support.

**Stay Consistent:** Remember that weight loss is a journey, and there may be ups and downs along the way. Stay consistent with your diet and exercise routine, and trust the process.

**Celebrate Your Successes:** Acknowledge and celebrate your achievements, no matter how small. This can help you stay motivated and focused on your goals.

# Chapter 5

## THE PRE-MAINTENANCE AND MAINTENANCE PHASES

## 1. Gradual reintroduction of carbohydrates in the Pre-Maintenance phase

**Increase Carb Intake:** Slowly increase your daily carbohydrate intake by about 10-20 grams per week. This can come from healthy sources like fruits, vegetables, and whole grains.

**Monitor Your Weight:** Continue to monitor your weight regularly. If you start gaining weight, reduce your carb intake slightly.

**Find Your Carb Balance:** Gradually increase your carb intake until you find a balance where you're maintaining your weight without feeling deprived or experiencing cravings.

**Stay Active:** Regular physical activity can help you manage your weight and improve your overall health.

**Stay Hydrated:** Drink plenty of water throughout the day to stay hydrated and support your metabolism.

**Listen to Your Body:** Pay attention to how your body responds to the increased carbs. If you experience any negative effects, such as bloating or cravings, adjust your carb intake accordingly.

**Healthy Carbohydrate Choices:** Focus on nutrient-dense carbohydrates like fruits, vegetables, legumes, and whole grains. Avoid processed and refined carbs.

## 2. Monitoring carbohydrate tolerance and finding the right balance for maintenance

**Gradual Reintroduction:** During the Pre-Maintenance phase, gradually increase your daily net carb intake by 10 grams each week. This will help you find your personal carb tolerance level.

**Monitor Your Weight:** Keep an eye on your weight and how your body feels as you increase your carb intake. If you start gaining weight or feeling sluggish, you may need to reduce your carb intake slightly.

**Listen to Your Body:** Pay attention to how different carb-rich foods affect your body. Some people may be able to tolerate certain carbs better than others.

**Keep a Food Diary:** Tracking your food intake can help you identify which foods and carb amounts work best for you.

**Stay Active:** Regular physical activity can help your body better manage carbs and maintain a healthy weight.

**Regularly Assess Your Progress:** Periodically reassess your carb intake and weight to ensure you're maintaining your desired weight and health goals.

**Consult a Healthcare Professional:** If you're unsure about how to proceed or need personalized advice, consider consulting with a healthcare professional or a dietitian who is familiar with low-carb diets like Atkins.

# 3. Strategies for long-term sustainability and weight maintenance

**Lifestyle Changes:** Focus on adopting sustainable lifestyle changes rather than short-term fixes. This includes making healthier food choices, being physically active, managing stress, and getting enough sleep.

**Regular Physical Activity:** Incorporate regular physical activity into your routine. Aim for a mix of cardiovascular exercise, strength training, and flexibility exercises. Find activities you enjoy to make it easier to stick with them.

**Mindful Eating:** Practice mindful eating by paying attention to your hunger and fullness cues. Avoid eating out of boredom or emotional reasons. Focus on enjoying your meals and savoring each bite.

**Regular Monitoring:** Continue to monitor your progress, including your weight, body measurements, and how you feel. This can help you stay on track and make adjustments if needed.

**Stay Hydrated:** Drink plenty of water throughout the day. Sometimes thirst is mistaken for hunger, so staying hydrated can help prevent overeating.

**Healthy Snacking:** Choose healthy snacks like fruits, vegetables, nuts, or yogurt. Avoid high-calorie, processed snacks that can contribute to weight gain.

**Balanced Diet:** Maintain a balanced diet that includes a variety of foods from all food groups. Include plenty of vegetables, fruits, whole grains, lean proteins, and healthy fats.

**Portion Control:** Be mindful of portion sizes to avoid overeating. Use smaller plates and bowls, and take your time eating to allow your body to feel full.

**Stay Flexible:** Allow yourself flexibility in your diet and exercise routine. It's okay to indulge occasionally, but try to get back on track quickly.

**Seek Support:** Stay connected with a support system, whether it's friends, family, or a support group. They can provide encouragement and accountability.

**Celebrate Your Successes:** Acknowledge and celebrate your achievements, no matter how small. This can help keep you motivated and positive.

**Professional Guidance:** Consider consulting with a healthcare professional or a registered dietitian for personalized advice and guidance.

# 4. Lifestyle considerations beyond diet (exercise, stress management, sleep)

**Exercise:** Regular physical activity is essential for maintaining a healthy weight, improving cardiovascular health, strengthening muscles and bones, and boosting mood and mental health. Aim for a mix of aerobic exercises (like walking, jogging, swimming) and strength training (like weight lifting or bodyweight exercises) for overall fitness.

**Stress Management:** Chronic stress can negatively impact health by affecting sleep, digestion, and mental health. Practicing stress-reducing techniques such as mindfulness meditation, yoga, deep breathing exercises, or engaging in hobbies can help manage stress levels.

**Sleep:** Quality sleep is vital for overall health and well-being. Poor sleep can contribute to weight gain, impaired cognitive function, and increased risk of chronic diseases. Establishing a regular sleep schedule, creating a relaxing bedtime routine, and ensuring a comfortable sleep environment can improve sleep quality.

# Chapter 6

# BEYOND THE BASICS: ADVANCED ATKINS STRATEGIES

## 1. Exploring advanced topics in the Atkins diet (intermittent fasting, carb cycling, targeted ketogenic diet)

**Intermittent Fasting (IF):** This eating pattern involves cycling between periods of eating and fasting. It can complement the Atkins diet by helping to regulate insulin levels and promote fat loss. Popular methods include 16/8 (fasting for 16 hours, eating within an 8-hour window) or 5:2 (eating normally for 5 days, and restricting calories for 2 non-consecutive days).

**Carb Cycling:** This technique involves alternating between high-carb and low-carb days. It can help prevent metabolic adaptation, where the body becomes more efficient at burning fewer calories. High-carb days can replenish glycogen stores, while low-carb days promote fat burning.

**Targeted Ketogenic Diet (TKD):** TKD allows for consuming a small amount of fast-digesting carbs, usually from sources like fruit or dextrose, around workouts. This provides a quick source of energy for exercise without significantly impacting ketosis.

## 2. Personalizing the Atkins diet for specific goals (athletic performance, metabolic health, medical conditions)

➢ **Athletic Performance:**

Ensure an adequate intake of protein to support muscle repair and growth.

Consider timing carbohydrate intake around workouts to optimize energy levels and performance.

Experiment with carb cycling, where you alternate between low-carb and higher-carb days based on training intensity and goals.

➢ **Metabolic Health:**

Focus on whole, nutrient-dense foods to support overall health and metabolism.

Monitor blood sugar levels regularly, especially if you have diabetes or insulin resistance.

Incorporate regular physical activity to improve insulin sensitivity and metabolic function.

> **Managing Medical Conditions:**

Consult with a healthcare professional before making significant dietary changes, especially if you have a medical condition.

Consider the potential impact of the Atkins diet on conditions such as diabetes, high blood pressure, and cholesterol levels.

Work with a healthcare provider to monitor any changes in symptoms or health markers and adjust your diet accordingly.

## 3. Resources for further learning and support (books, websites, communities)

> **Books:**

The Vegetable Gardener's Container Bible by Edward C. Smith - A comprehensive guide to container gardening with vegetables, herbs, and fruits.

Coloring Mandalas by Susanne F. Fincher - A book that explores the therapeutic benefits of coloring mandalas.

The MacroNutrient Diet Cookbook by Amanda Bryant - A cookbook with macro-friendly recipes and meal planning tips.

The New Atkins for a New You by Eric C. Westman, Stephen D. Phinney, and Jeff S. Volek - A guide to the Atkins diet with updated information and meal plans.

> **Websites:**

**Balcony Gardening:** Check out resources like the Royal Horticultural Society's website (rhs.org.uk), which offers tips and guides for balcony gardening.

**Coloring Techniques:** Websites like Color-Matters (color-matters.com) provide information on color theory and its effects.

**Macro Tracking:** MyFitnessPal (myfitnesspal.com) and Cronometer (cronometer.com) are popular apps for tracking macros and calories.

**Atkins Diet:** The official Atkins website (atkins.com) offers a wealth of information, including recipes, meal plans, and community support.

> **Communities:**

**Gardening:** Join online communities like the subreddit r/gardening or the forums on GardenWeb (gardenweb.com) to connect with other gardeners.

**Coloring:** Look for coloring groups on social media platforms like Facebook, where members share tips, techniques, and finished works.

Macro Tracking: Join groups on Facebook or Reddit focused on macro tracking and the Atkins diet for support and advice from others following similar paths.

> **Local Resources:**

Consider joining a local gardening club or attending gardening workshops at a nearby botanical garden or nursery for hands-on learning and community support.

Look for local art classes or workshops that focus on coloring or other artistic techniques for a creative outlet and potential community connections.

# 4. Conclusion and final tips for success on the Atkins diet

**Stay Committed:** Remember, the Atkins diet is a lifestyle change, not a quick fix. Stay committed to your health and wellness goals.

**Monitor Progress:** Continue to track your food intake, weight, and measurements to stay on track and make adjustments as needed.

**Gradual Reintroduction of Carbohydrates:** As you move into the Pre-Maintenance phase, gradually reintroduce carbohydrates to find your personal carb balance for maintenance.

**Focus on Whole Foods:** Choose whole, nutrient-dense foods to support your health and provide sustained energy.

**Stay Hydrated:** Drink plenty of water throughout the day to stay hydrated and support your body's functions.

**Physical Activity:** Incorporate regular physical activity into your routine to support weight loss and overall health.

**Mindful Eating:** Pay attention to your body's hunger and fullness cues to prevent overeating.

**Seek Support:** Join a community or find a support system to stay motivated and accountable.

**Celebrate Your Success:** Acknowledge and celebrate your achievements, no matter how small. Every step forward is a step closer to your goals.

**Consult with a Professional:** If you have any questions or concerns, consult with a healthcare professional or a registered dietitian to ensure you're following the Atkins diet safely and effectively.